The *GOLF Magazine*
Golf Fitness
Handbook

Other titles in the series

The *GOLF Magazine* Course Management Handbook
The *GOLF Magazine* Mental Golf Handbook

The *GOLF Magazine* Golf Fitness Handbook

Gary Wiren, Ph.D.
PGA Master Professional
and the Editors of *GOLF Magazine*

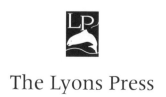

The Lyons Press

Copyright © 1999 by Gary Wiren

First Lyons Press edition—1999

Printed in the United States of America
Design and composition by Compset, Inc.

10 9 8 7 6 5 4 3 2 1

Library of Congress Cataloging-in-Publication Data

Wiren, Gary.
   The Golf magazine golf fitness handbook/Gary Wiren and the editors of Golf magazine. —1st Lyons Press ed.
      p. cm.
   ISBN 1-55821-808-4 (pbk.)
      1. Golf—Training. 2. Physical fitness. I. Golf magazine. II. Title
      GV979.T68W57 1999
   613.7'4—dc21   99-18221
                                                CIP

Contents

FOREWORD

At *Golf Magazine* we use two methods to determine the content of each issue: surveys and guts. In the survey method, questionnaires are sent to thousands of subscribers, asking—among other things—what topics they enjoy most and which kinds of articles they prefer. In the guts method, we editors simply use our intuition as kindred, hopelessly addicted golfers.

But no matter which method we use, the number one request is always for the same thing: instruction. "Give us more instruction" has been the mandate from our readers ever since the magazine began publishing, forty years ago. The reason is simple: A golfer is happiest when his game is improving.

Recently, however, we've learned a couple of things about how to present our instruction. First, you like it short and sweet. After all, most of the current population were raised on television, sound bites, and quick delivery of information—from beepers to e-mail. More than ever, we like our messages short and to the point.

And the "to the point" part is just as important as the "short" part. For the last decade or so, the most popular portion of *Golf Magazine* has been the buff-colored section, "Private Lessons," which brings together custom-tailored instruction for five different kinds of golfers: low handicappers, high handicappers, short but straight hitters, long but crooked hitters, and senior golfers. In this way, we're able to speak more personally with our readers and help them more individually with their games.

Why am I telling you all this? Because the same kind of thinking went into the book that is now in your hands. When the people at the Lyons Press came to talk to us about a partnership in golf-book publishing, we gave them our mantra for success: instruction, succinct and focused. The result is the *Golf Magazine* series of guides, each written concisely, edited mercilessly, and dedicated entirely to one key aspect of playing the game.

Each *Golf Magazine* guide assembles a wealth of great advice in a package small enough to carry in your golf bag. We hope you'll use these pages to raise your game to a whole new level.

—George Peper
Editor-in-Chief
Golf Magazine

The *GOLF Magazine* Golf Fitness Handbook

Introduction

It's hard to imagine any competitive sport today in which the participants do not physically train for their event; even table tennis and chess players do. *Training is an absolute necessity if participants expect to perform at their highest level.* Yet golfers have been slow to recognize the seemingly obvious benefits of training. Golf professionals from a previous generation were the victims of "old wives' tales" about the negative implications of building muscles for golf. Not so today. That's why you see official PGA fitness trainers on the Tour, college teams that have training regimes, mini-Tour players working out regularly, and national amateur squads with strict physical training programs.

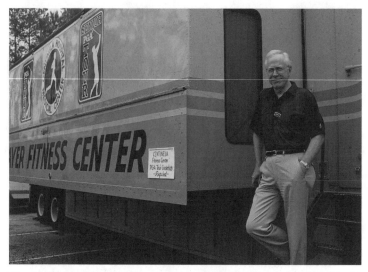

The golfing public started taking more notice of training specifically for golf when the PGA Tour fitness trainers appeared.

The average amateur golfer, however, is still trying to *buy* better performance through exotic clubs, "hot golf balls," and secrets from gurus. Certainly proper equipment and good instruction do help. But you can't win the Indianapolis 500 in a Volkswagen. And you can't make the golf ball respond as you'd like it to if your body can't generate speed or provide control. The "average player" may be limited to "average" by a poorly conditioned body: one that is either too weak, too fat, too inflexible, or all three. So awaken to the reality that *your technique will always be limited by your body's ability to per-*

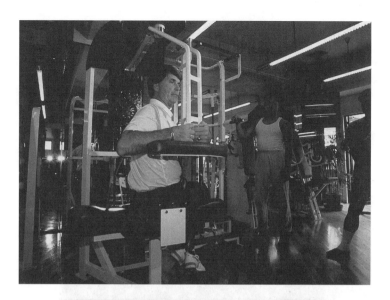

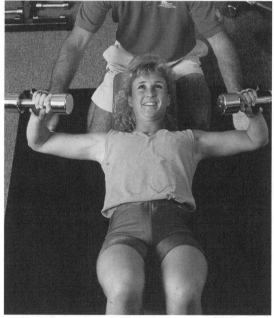

Working out in the training center is a part of every major college golf program as well as for those players competing on the mini-Tour.

form. Let's be honest: Golf is an athletic event. Other factors being equal, the trained athlete beats the untrained one on a regular basis.

Besides performance enhancement, there are at least three other very good reasons to train for golf:

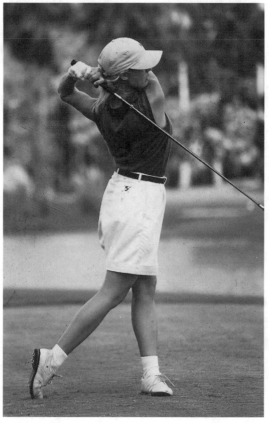

A dynamic full-motion golf swing is a true athletic move.

1. *You will be less likely to sustain injury,* and if you do have an injury, you will recuperate much more quickly.

2. *You will increase your golfing longevity.* Well-conditioned golfers can maintain pleasurable golfing skills into their seventies, eighties, and even nineties, which makes golf "the game of a lifetime."

3. Finally, the greatest benefit to training for golf is that you are also training for life. If your desire to improve your golf handicap can motivate you to adopt a more active, healthier lifestyle, not only will your golf get better, but so will the quality of your living. *You'll feel better, look better, and play better.* That's quite a combination . . . if you follow through with it.

PROMISE

How can this book help you cash in on the promises just described? Hopefully, those potential rewards are sufficient to motivate you to action. Oh, it will take effort, but the results are truly worth it. (I say that from a lifetime of personal experience.) So, if somewhere deep inside you there is an honest desire to be a better golfer, then becoming fit for golf is a goal you definitely need to pursue. Why? Because it can make a huge difference in performance. This book can give you the right information to make that difference.

Knowing the demands of a busy lifestyle and realizing that unrealistic expectations often lead to quitting and failure, I have deliberately limited the number of exercises and time for exercising to twenty to forty minutes per workout. To help with the time problem, you are even shown how to build exercise into your life without taking any extra time. Material is offered that ranges from nutrition considerations that are golf specific, to managing your life to protect you from back trauma. So choose from these golf exercise programs what best suits your schedule. Balance them between strength, flexibility, and endurance, and include the whole body. Let's get started—it all starts with warm-up.

Warm-Up

The Necessity of Warm-up

When you walk to the first tee without having warmed up, you can expect to be greeted by muscles, tendons, and ligaments that are cold, inflexible, and unforgiving. You are asking (almost begging) for injury or poor performance. Too many times, I have seen the man who leaves the locker room, strolls to the first tee, takes out the driver, makes two swings at a cigarette butt or broken tee on the ground, considers that to be his warm-up, and asks, "How much we playin' for?" Then there is the woman (on ladies' day) whose version of a warm-up prior to the shotgun start consists of a cup of coffee, a danish, and lots of conversation followed by her uninspired practice swings when she arrives at the designated tee location. This is not an adequate warm-up. It encourages injury and discourages good performance.

Compare these examples to other sports. In football the players are on the field forty-five minutes ahead of the kick-off doing calisthenics and run-

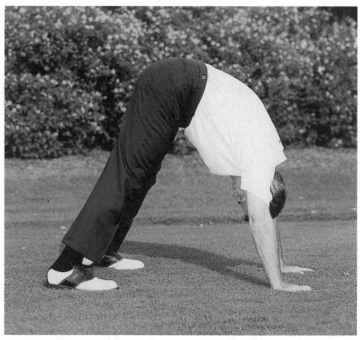

This is a great hamstring and back stretch that can be done in the locker room, on the practice range, or on the first tee prior to play.

ning through skill drills to warm up. In basketball (men's or women's) the warm-up starts about thirty minutes prior to the center jump. Then there is baseball (or softball), in which it seems the pre-game warm-up lasts almost as long as the game itself. All of these rituals are performed in order to warm up. Why do golfers think they are exempt from the laws of physiology?

Fortunately, the golf warm-up can be done much more quickly than what I've described in these other sports. But just because you aren't tackling someone, jumping for a rebound, or circling the bases *don't think that the golf swing isn't a physically demanding movement that needs its own specific warm-up.* The following pages will give you options to accomplish that physiological need.

Three Warm-Up Options

Home or Locker Room Warm-up

Taking six minutes to do some stretching before leaving for the course, or in the locker room after you arrive, is a great way to start preparation for your round. The following stretches are suggested for an effective golf warm-up before you get to the practice tee.

Stretch to Ceiling: Interlock your fingers and extend both arms overhead with your palms toward the ceiling. Tilt your head back while looking at your hands. Rise up on your toes as you stretch overhead. Hold the stretch for ten seconds. Repeat three times.

Muscles used: Arms, neck, shoulders, and calves.

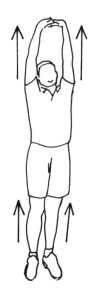

Back Scratch: Stand upright and place one hand in the center of your back. Pull down on the bent elbow with the opposite hand; hold for ten seconds. Repeat three times on each side.

Muscles used: Triceps, forearms, and rotator cuff.

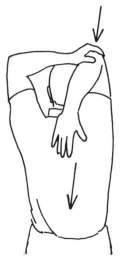

Side Bends: Interlock your fingers and extend both arms overhead. Bend to one side by pulling slowly with one arm toward the ground. Keep your elbows on plane with the body. Hold the stretch for ten seconds. Repeat three times on each side. *Muscles used:* Obliques, upper back, and shoulders.

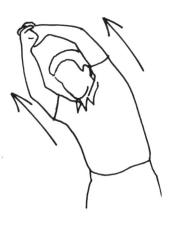

Wall Touches: While standing with your back about one foot away from a wall, slowly turn your torso until you can place one or both palms flat on the wall. Try to keep your hips facing forward and your knees slightly bent. Hold for ten seconds. Repeat three times on each side. *Muscles used:* Abdominals, obliques, and lower back.

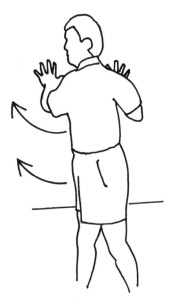

Standing Hamstring Stretch: Stand on one leg. Slowly raise your opposite foot close to thigh height. Rest your heel on a stable object, such as a bench. Interlock your fingers, then slowly stretch forward toward the elevated foot. Hold for ten seconds. Repeat three times on each leg.
Muscles used: Hamstrings, calves, and lower back.

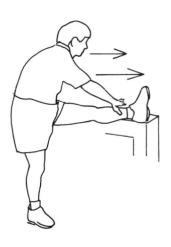

Bench Lunges: Stand two to three feet away from a stable bench and place your hands on your hips. Raise one leg and place your foot flat on the bench. Slowly shift your weight over the forward leg. Don't allow the front knee to extend out over your toes. Repeat five times on each leg.
Muscles used: Hips, quadriceps, and hamstrings.

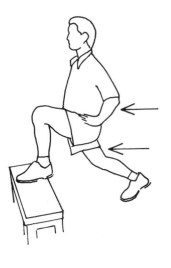

Golf Car Stretching

The golf car can be a valuable piece of stretching equipment as well as a means of transportation. If you haven't done the home or locker room warm-up exercises, you may wish to do the following stretches, utilizing the golf car, before you tee off. It is a good idea to repeat some of these stretches during the round if you feel yourself becoming tight or fatigued.

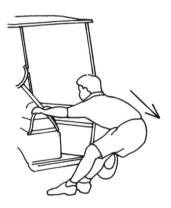

Lower Back Stretch: While standing facing a golf car from about one foot away, grab the arm guard with both hands. Fully extend your arms. Slowly bend your knees and sit back away from the car until you feel a stretch in the lower back. Hold for ten seconds. Repeat three times.

Muscles used: Lower back and shoulders.

Rear Shoulder Stretch:
Stand at a 90-degree angle
to the golf car. Reach
across your body with
your outside hand and
grab the roof post at shoulder height. Slowly turn
away from the car, stretching your rear shoulder
and back muscles. Do two
repetitions and hold the
stretch for ten seconds.
Repeat with your other
arm while facing the op-
posite direction.
Muscles used: Rear shoulders, upper back, and
torso.

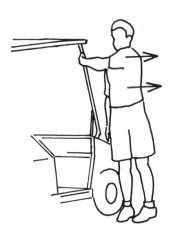

Front Shoulder Stretch:
Stand facing away from
the golf car, reach back,
and grab the roof post
with one hand. Keep your
hand at shoulder height
with the palm facing out.

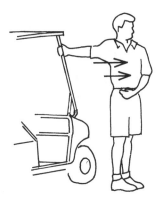

Slowly turn away from your hand holding the post. Hold for ten seconds. Repeat twice. Repeat with the opposite arm.

Muscles used: Chest, shoulders, biceps, forearms, and torso.

Middle Back and Hamstring Stretch: Hold on to the roof post with one hand. Slowly lean away, keeping one leg extended out with the toes pointed up. Grab the toes with one hand to stretch your hamstring; sit back to stretch the middle back. Hold for ten seconds. Repeat on the other side.

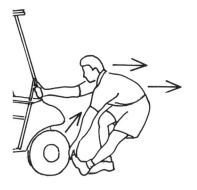

Muscles used: Hamstrings, calves, shoulders, and middle back.

Gravity Drop: Stand with both feet on the golf car floor, balancing on the forward part of each foot. Hold on to the roof for support and let your heels drop down toward the ground. Slowly lower and raise your heels. Repeat ten times.

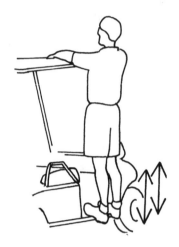

Muscles used: Achilles tendon and calves.

Golf Car Lunges: Rest a golf club across your upper back, standing approximately two to three feet away from a golf car. Raise one leg and place your foot flat on the floor. Slowly shift your weight over the forward leg. Don't let your front knee extend out over your toes. Repeat three times on each leg.

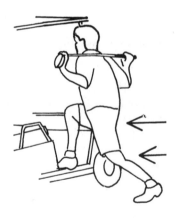

Muscles used: Hips, quadriceps, and hamstrings.

Should you find yourself arriving just in time to tee off and no time to do either the golf car stretching or the locker room warm-up, then use the following "No-Ball Warm-Up." You can fit in some of the locker room and golf car stretches while you play the opening holes.

The "No-Ball Warm-Up" on the First Tee

Tour professional golfers arrive at the course allowing one to one and a half hours to prepare before

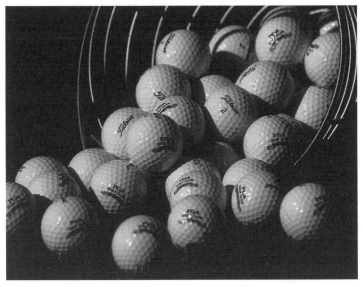

Hitting balls before play is an advantage that shouldn't be over-looked.

hitting the first tee shot. This provides adequate time to get their equipment organized, do some of the physical warm-up exercises just described, a little ball hitting, short game practice, and putting. Ideally, that's what we all should do. But if you are like most golfers, rarely are you so fortunate. Frequently, you come to the course allowing just enough time to change shoes, check in at the pro shop, and head to the first tee.

Since you seldom have the luxury of arriving an hour before you tee off, and if you didn't do any home or locker room stretches, what can you do when you find yourself on the tee without having done any exercises or hit any shots to warm up? One recommendation is for you to take at least ninety seconds to perform a six-step "No Ball Warm-Up." Here is how you do it:

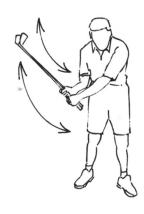

Step 1 (20 seconds): Take your two heaviest clubs—i.e., sand wedge and pitching wedge— and hold them together in a semi-baseball grip. Feel the heaviness of the two combined and begin making small swings, hands traveling first to hip height, then shoulder height, gradually building up the length to a full swing. The extra weight will not only help you stretch but also will promote a better tempo and true swinging motion. If at any time during these stretches, particularly the next five, you feel a sharp pull of pain, stop and reduce the stress load in the position you are attempting.

Step 2 (20 seconds): Select the club you are going to use from the first tee (probably a driver or #3 wood). Standing vertically, place the club behind your back in the crooks of your elbows and turn a total of 180 degrees, (including back and through swings). Get your abdomen to face the target at the finish and let your weight naturally transfer from your rear foot to your forward foot.

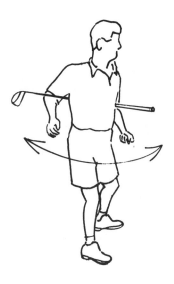

Step 3 (15 seconds): Bend
forward from the hips as
though addressing the
ball. With this forward tilt
of the spine maintained,
repeat the total of 180-
degree turns, allowing
your weight to shift from
over your rear leg to over
your forward leg; again
you should be "tummy
to the target," looking at
your target, not the
ground, at the finish.

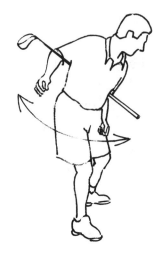

Step 4 (15 seconds):
Standing vertically,
place the club across
your shoulders and be-
hind your neck, grasp-
ing it with the right and
left hand spread beyond
shoulder's width. Turn
180 degrees; 90 back
and 90 through. Use the
same lower body finish
as before.

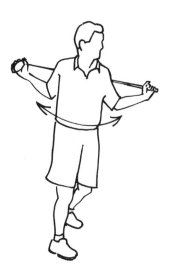

Step 5 (15 seconds): Keeping the club in the same position, tilt your spine forward to assume your address position and repeat the exercise. Face the target at the finish.

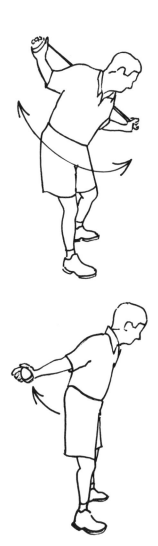

Step 6 (15 seconds): From the previous position, drop the club behind your back to hip height, keeping your thumbs hooked around the shaft. Raise your arms behind you and make 180-degree turns with your body, always finishing with the weight off the rear foot and on your forward foot. The higher you raise your arms the greater the stretch.

That's eighty seconds of stretching. Allowing ten seconds more to change clubs and positions, and you have a ninety-second no-ball warm-up. Now take a few easy practice swings, gradually increasing your speed until you have reached a comfortable, effective rate; *not your hardest* but your most

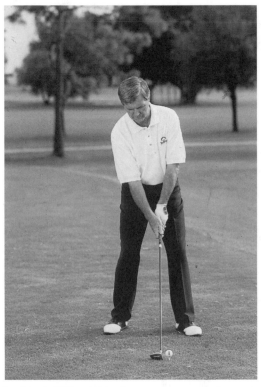

After the No-Ball Warm-Up, focus on a good aim and setup.

effective. Tee the ball, go through your preshot routine, and swing with the effort of the last comfortable but aggressive full practice swing. *You'll be starting your round with the knowledge and confidence that you have had an adequate warm-up to hit a respectable drive.*

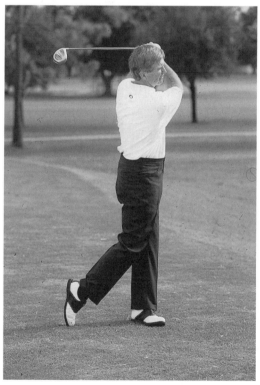

Then, "make your very best swing," not your hardest hit.

Combinations of any of the three warm-up options just recommended can be used. Obviously, hitting practice shots on the practice range prior to play is desirable to establish your feel and rehearse your routine as well as to stretch and warm your muscles, ligaments, and tendons. The important thing is to warm up in a way that will help you develop the feel for your swing and discourage any chance of injuring yourself.

Key Fitness Components

Flexibility

When golfers think of hitting the ball farther, they immediately relate it to physical strength. But strength without the range of motion needed to apply it is of limited value. Power is the result of applying force over a given distance in a specified time. If one has a body with a trunk that can barely turn or knees that hardly flex, arms that refuse to extend, a spine that won't stay tilted, and wrists that resist cocking, the answer to better performance is to *increase flexibility*!

Stretching to increase range of motion and maximize one's power is the hottest, most "in" part of golf exercise among the game's top players. It is an absolute neces-

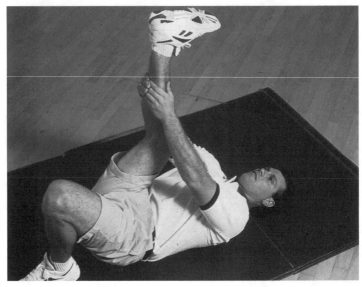

This hamstring stretch will help reduce potential back problems, thus allowing you to make a strong rotary movement in your swing.

sity for longevity in the game, and one of the surest antidotes for the prevention of injury.

When performing flexibility exercises there are a few important imperatives to follow:

1. Warm up before beginning stretching exercises by performing some total body movement like jumping jacks or jogging in place.

2. Always do stretching slowly. Never bounce to increase range of motion.

3. Don't push your pain level. Distinguish between slight discomfort and sharp pain.

4. Breathe naturally. Exhale as you do your stretch, and continue breathing as you hold the position.

5. To get the most out of a stretching exercise, go to your comfortable limit, relax, then go just a bit farther.

6. Hold your stretch positions from ten to thirty seconds and occasionally longer depending on the exercise. Generally longer is better.

7. Inhale deeply through your nose and exhale through your nose or mouth.

8. Make it a habit of taking stretch breaks during the day, such as stretching when you are just standing waiting for the bus, a plane, in a line at the store, by your desk, in the kitchen or front room; literally wherever you happen to be.

Using the stretches that have been described before you play will provide you with many benefits. It will increase your blood supply to muscles, ligaments, and tendons; elongate muscle tissue; reduce tension; and improve movement around the joints. *These kinds of benefits, which help prevent injury and improve performance, should encourage everyone to do some warm-up related to stretching before play.* For long-term improved golf performance, however, you need a regular program of stretching that is done more frequently than just on days you play. Here is a suggested collection of simple home workout stretching exercises.

Regular Flexibility Home Workout

The following exercises should be done every day to increase flexibility in your trunk and lower extremities. If every day is not possible, then at least every other day is recommended for sustained improvement.

Tuck Roll: While lying flat on your back, pull both knees into your chest with interlocked fingers. Slowly make small rocking motions back and forth between the upper and lower back. Repeat ten times. *Muscles used:* Gluteus, lower back, and shoulders.

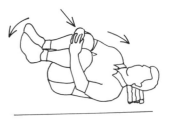

Double Toe Tug: While lying flat on your back, elevate both feet into the air. Hood a towel over your toes and slowly pull downward. Push your heels upward to increase the stretch. Repeat five times. *Muscles used:* Hamstrings and calves.

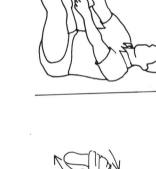

Single Toe Cross-over: While lying flat on your back, bend both knees. Raise one foot in the air, hooking a towel over your toes. Pull the foot toward the opposite shoulder. Hold for ten seconds. Repeat three times on each leg. *Muscles used:* Hips and gluteus.

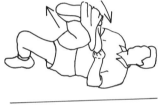

Hip Extension Stretch:
While lying flat on your back, bend both knees. Cross one foot over the opposite knee, then slowly rotate your torso toward the same side as your upper leg. Keep the shoulders flat as you hold the stretch for ten seconds. Repeat three times on each side.

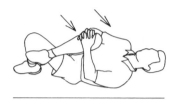

Muscles used: Hip flexors, lower back, and torso.

Trunk Rotation: While lying flat on your back, bend both knees. Cross one foot over the opposite knee. Slowly rotate your torso toward the opposite side of your upper leg. Use your opposite hand to pull. Repeat three times on each side.

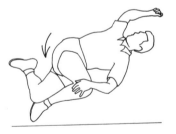

Muscles used: Lower back, abdominals, and torso.

Fitness Center Flexibility

Lower Body

The following six-exercise stretching workout is a bit more advanced and may be easier to do at a fitness center. Any of the home exercises could also be incorporated. Hold each of these stretches for ten seconds. Apply consistent pressure during every stretch. Do not bounce. Attempt to exhale your breath out through your mouth as you perform each stretch. This first group of six is for your lower and midbody.

Wall Double-Leg Stretch: Lying flat on your back, place your heels on the wall, keeping the legs fully extended. Slowly pull your toes downward, without bending knees. Alternate feet. Repeat ten times.
Muscles used: Gastrocnemius, hamstrings, and lower back.

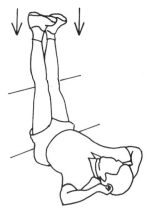

Wall Single Leg/Heel on Toe: Lying flat on your back with your seat close to the wall and legs fully extended, place your heels against the wall. Slowly place one heel on the opposite toe. Apply additional resistance by pressing lightly on your front thigh. Repeat three times. Switch legs.

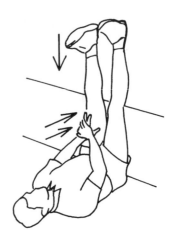

Muscles used: Hamstrings and achilles tendon.

Wall Alternate Instep Pull: Lying flat on your back, place your heels on the wall. Grab the instep of one foot with your same side hand. Press your heel up toward the ceiling. Repeat three times. Switch legs.

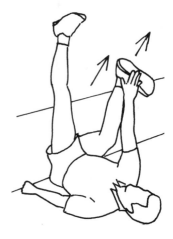

Muscles used: Gluteals, calves, and hamstrings.

Wall Figure-4 Stretch: Lying flat on your back, bend both knees until they are in a 90-degree angle. Then, cross one foot over your opposite knee. Pull down on your toes with one hand while pushing on one knee with your opposite hand. You should feel stretching in the back of your leg. Repeat three times. Switch legs.

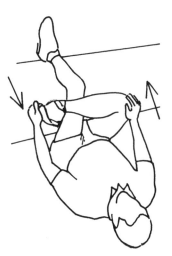

Muscles used: Gluteals and lower back.

Bench Single-Leg Stretch: Sit up tall on a bench. Place one leg out in front of you, the other flat on the floor. Interlock your fingers and slowly stretch forward. Repeat three times and hold each stretch at the maximum extension. Switch legs.

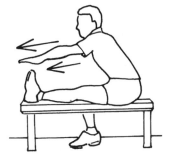

Muscles used: Hamstrings, calves, lower back, and shoulders.

Bench Ankle Grab: Place one knee on a bench and put your other foot flat on the floor in front of you. The toes of the front foot must be in front of your bent knee. Slowly bend the knee that's on the bench and reach back and grab your ankle with the same side hand. Slowly pull your ankle forward. Repeat three times. Switch legs.

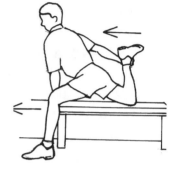

Muscles used: Quadriceps, hip flexors, and lower back.

Upper Body

For an upper-body flexibility workout at home or at the fitness center, use the following exercises that have already been cited as part of a home or locker room warm-up or golf car stretching routine: **Stretch to ceiling, back scratch, wall touches, side bends, rear shoulder stretch, and front shoulder stretch.** You can utilize these same upper-body exercises and any of the other home stretching or warm-up exercises at the fitness center by inserting them in between the exercises in your strength workout. For example, if you use a back extension machine for strength, you might insert a thirty-second wall touch for flexibility. Matching a stretching exercise to the muscle group you have just worked on for strength keeps you flexible while building additional strength. *The combination of strength and flexibility is the secret for achieving power.*

Strength

The power in the golf swing comes from muscular action, which drives the torso, limbs, and eventually the club to deliver a blow to the ball. It takes an estimated 60 pounds of muscular mass to create a clubhead speed of 100 m.p.h. (240-yard drive). Therefore, *doing exercises to build stronger muscles can definitely increase your potential for distance.* The amount of gain will depend greatly upon where you start. If you are already strong and have good muscle tone, the gains from strength training alone may be small. But if you are in poor muscular condition and have low levels of strength, those gains could be quite large. There is one caveat pertaining to any predictions in performance gain: *You can expect maximum positive results only if you do the prescribed suggested exercises regularly and correctly.*

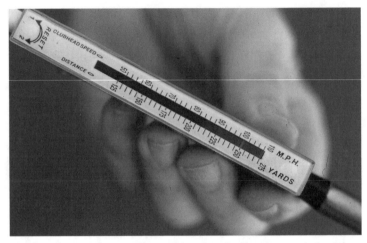

Clubhead speed, as measured by the device shown, is largely a product of a strength and flexibility that is specific to golf, for which you can train.

Here are some important principles you should be aware of before embarking on a strength-building program.

- *It is never too late to get stronger.* Recent research at Tufts University documents strength increases from 10 percent to 226 percent in subjects whose average ages were in their sixties and seventies. Also at Harvard, significant strength gains were demonstrated in a group of both men and women ranging in age from eighty-six to ninety-six.

- *You can't get stronger without stressing your muscular system.* This stress can come from providing a resistance, which could consist of more weight, more repetitions, or more tension, as in an isometric (static) exercise, or by moving the load with more speed.

- *An alternative way to add repetitions is to do a second or third set.* This can be done for any group of muscles on which you wish to focus.

- *Don't go too fast.* Add weight, repetition, or speed gradually and comfortably. The biggest mistake a motivated person can make is to think that two weeks of exercise will undo what has happened to the body over the previous twenty years. Be patient! Go slowly and do it regularly!

- *Rest days in between strength-building days are essential.* Training breaks the muscles fibers down and rest gives them the opportunity to build back up and grow.

- *Don't hold your breath during a lift.* It increases the blood pressure, lowers the heart rate, and can cause blackout. Exhale during the exertion portion and inhale before completion of the repetition.

- *Movements should be steady, not jerky.* Don't choose a load that is so heavy that you lose your good form.

- *Work the large muscles before the small muscles.* Large muscle activity can assist in warming up the smaller ones and they fatigue less rapidly.

At-Home Strength Training

For strength training I recommend using a weight resistance that will allow you to successfully complete at least ten repetitions. When you can complete fifteen repetitions, add weight and reduce the reps to ten again. Dumbbells or hand weights are suggested, but water bottles, cartons of sand, or similar weighted objects can be used. Working out three to four days per week on strength training is recommended. One hard day of strength training per week might maintain your present level, two days would give you some increase, but three to four days of a vigorous (but not intensive) program has been shown to be the most beneficial.

There are also specialized golf strength and flexibility training products that can be used at home.* One of the simplest and most useful for golf is a hand gripper. The hands are the only connection between the power source, your body, and the delivery system, the club. Strong golf starts with strong hands. This is true even more so for control of the club than it is for distance. Home golf training equipment is readily available and quite effective, providing you actually use it.

---

*See the reference at the end of the book.

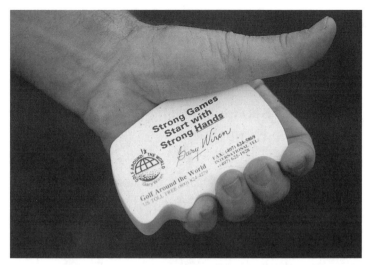

A hand gripper may be one of the least expensive but most beneficial exercise aids you could own.

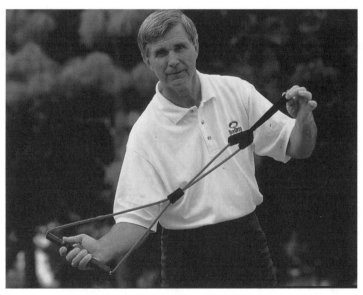

Rubber tubing has gained popularity among athletes for resistance training in many sports, including golf.

Upper Body

Wall Side Raises: From a standing position, place your back against the wall and spread your feet comfortably apart. Start with your hands at hip height and slowly raise your arms vertically until they are at shoulder height. Lower to the starting position. Repeat ten times.

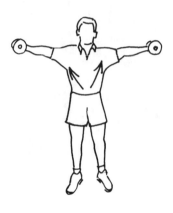

Muscles used: Shoulders, forearms, and wrists.

Wall Shoulder Shrugs: From a standing position, place your back against the wall and spread your feet comfortably apart. Start with your hands at hip height and slowly raise your shoulders vertically toward your ears. Return to the starting position. Do not rotate your shoulders

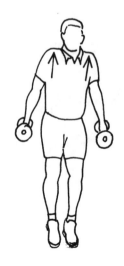

or bend your arms at the elbows. Repeat ten times.
Muscles used: Trapezius, upper back, and shoulders.

Wall Vertical Raise/ Horizontal Press: From a standing position, place your back against the wall and spread your feet comfortably apart. Start with your hands in front of your thighs. Slowly raise both hands to your chin, keeping your elbows higher than the hands. Now press your hands straight out in front of you at shoulder level until fully extended. Slowly lower your hands to the starting position. Repeat ten times.

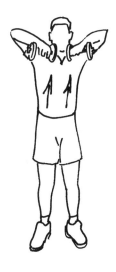

Muscles used: Forearms, triceps, trapezius, and upper back.

Seated Forearm Curls and Reverse Curls: From a seated position, rest the back of your forearm on the top of your thigh with the wrist extended beyond your knee. Slowly raise and lower the weight by flexing and extending the wrist. Repeat ten times, then switch arms.

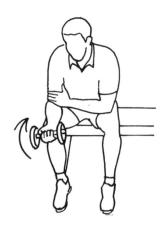

Muscles used: Forearm flexors and extensors.

One Arm Rows: Bend forward, placing one knee and one hand on a bench, while keeping your back flat. Let your hand with the weight extend toward the ground, then slowly raise your arm until the el-

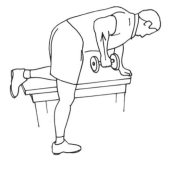

bow is flexed at a 90-degree angle. Slowly lower the weight to the starting position. Repeat ten times. *Muscles used:* Latissimus dorsi, triceps, and rear deltoids.

Weighted Side Bends: Stand upright with one hand on top of your head and the other hand beside your hip. Place your feet shoulder-width apart. Slowly bend from side to side, keeping your body in a straight plane. *Do not bend forward.* Repeat ten times on each side.

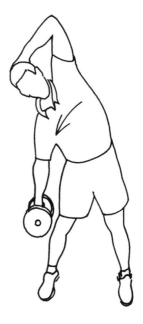

Muscles used: Obliques, lower back, and abdominals.

Lower Body and Abdominals

Calf Raises/Double and Single: (Double) Stand facing a wall with your feet shoulder-width apart. Slowly raise up on your toes until your heels are fully extended off the floor. Repeat for twenty-five repetitions. (Single) Place one foot behind your other heel. Slowly raise up on your toes until your heel is fully extended off the floor. Repeat fifteen times on each leg.
Muscles used: Calves and achilles tendon.

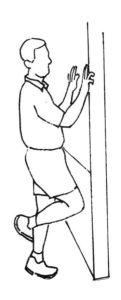

Air Bench: From a standing position, place your back against the wall and spread your feet comfortably apart. Bend your knees and position your feet away from the wall two to three feet. Your

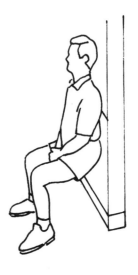

weight should be balanced equally on both heels. Hold your air bench for at least thirty seconds. Repeat five to ten times.

Muscles used: Thighs, hamstrings, and buttocks.

Bent-knee Crunches: Lie on your back and bend your knees to 90 degrees while keeping your feet flat on the floor. Lift your legs in the air, keeping your knees bent at a 90-degree angle. Cross your hands over your chest or support your head with your hands lightly holding your ears. Slowly raise your upper body toward your knees. Keep your elbows pointed at your knees during the exercise. Repeat twenty times.

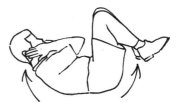

Muscles used: Abdominal and hip flexors.

Crossover Crunches: Lie on your back with your knees bent so that your heels are flat on the floor. Cross one leg over the other so that one ankle is resting on your opposite knee. Cross your hands over your chest and slowly raise your upper body towards the crossed knee. Avoid putting pressure on your neck by keeping your eyes on the ceiling. Repeat twenty times.

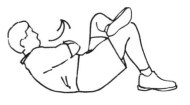

Muscles used: External obliques and abdominals.

Bent-knee Raises: Lie on your back with your knees bent so that your heels are flat on the floor. Keeping your knees bent, slowly raise your knees up toward your chest, then return. Control the move-

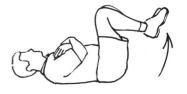

ment in both directions, trying not to use momentum. Repeat twenty-five times.
Muscles used: Lower abdominals.

Prone Trunk Raises: Lie on your stomach with your legs together, fully extended and your hands at your sides or crossed over your chest. Slowly raise your upper body toward the ceiling keeping your lower body on the floor. Lift only your upper body. Repeat fifteen times.

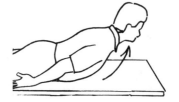

Muscles used: Lower lumbar.

Fitness Center Strength Training

Going to a fitness center gives you the opportunity to work with more sophisticated machines that can isolate specific muscle groups and accurately control weight loads. Utilize the professional staff there to help you assess your current level of fitness and plan a program to meet your goals. Once this is accomplished they will take you through the routine

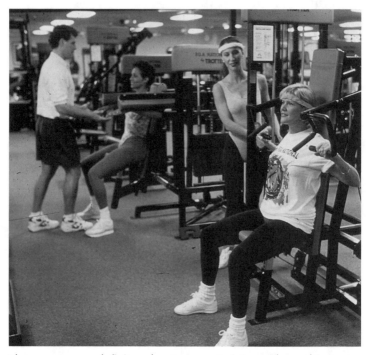

There are some definite advantages to training with machines at a fitness center.

and show you how to use each machine correctly. There are fundamental principles for exercising (some of which have been mentioned) that when followed can make a great deal of difference in your progress. The staff should review these with you.

The fitness center exercises are recommended specifically for golf, although a local trainer may modify the program after making a personal assessment. In general, it is suggested that you complete at least one set of ten repetitions for each exercise. As you become stronger, add a second and third set of eight to fifteen repetitions. For a more intense workout and greater cardiovascular fitness, you might occasionally do several exercises in a row without resting in between. This will get your heart rate up and put more demand on your lungs. Adding your stretching in between the strength sets will do the same, only to a lesser degree.

Don't hesitate to call upon the staff to help you with technique and some of the details of resistance training with machines, such as seeing that your seat adjustments are correct for your height and that your rhythm on the lift and return are correct.

Upper Body

Chest Press: Using an upright or prone chest press machine, position your body so that your hands and chest muscles are in alignment. Slowly press your hands away from your chest until your arms are about 90 percent extended. Do not lock your elbows. Slowly lower the weight back to your starting position. Repeat ten times. Be sure to exhale when pushing the weight. *Muscles used:* Chest and triceps.

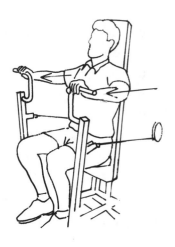

Lateral Raise: Select a lateral raise machine and align yourself in a position so that your forearms rest on the arm pads. Slowly raise the weight up to

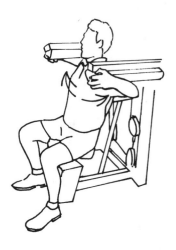

shoulder height. Avoid lifting the weight above your shoulders. Slowly lower the weight back to your starting position. Repeat ten times.

Muscles used: Deltoids and trapezius.

Triceps Press: Using a triceps press machine, align yourself in a position that keeps your feet flat on the floor. Select a grip with your palms facing each other. Keep your elbows close to your side and slowly press the weight until your arms are 90 percent extended. Slowly allow the weight to return to your starting position. Repeat ten times.

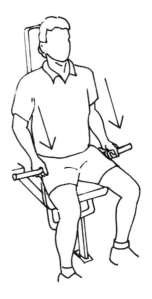

Muscles used: Triceps and forearms.

Cable-cross Chest Fly: Stand in the middle of a cable-cross machine holding a handle in each hand. Slowly bring your hands together in front of you. Remain stationary, then slowly return your hands to their starting position. Lean your body slightly forward at the waist. Your feet should be at least shoulder-width apart. Repeat ten times.

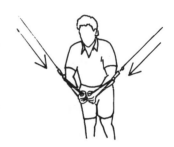

Muscles used: Chest, shoulders, and biceps.

Isolation Cable-cross Curls: Stand up straight in the middle of a cable-cross machine holding a handle in each hand. Slowly bring your hands in toward your ears. Keep your elbows pointed out as you squeeze your upper arms. Slowly return your hands

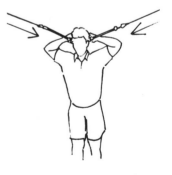

to the starting position. Repeat ten times.

Muscles used: Shoulders and biceps.

Single-arm Cable-cross Extensions: Stand parallel to a cable cross machine. Hold a handle in your hand that is away from the machine. Position your feet shoulder-width apart and slowly pull your arm across your body, pulling your hand down from your shoulder to the opposite pocket. Keep your arm straight during the exercise. Slowly return to the starting position. Repeat ten times with each arm.

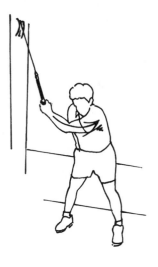

Muscles used: Upper back and shoulders.

Note: If a cable cross machine is not available at your fitness center, the following machines are recommended; *chest fly, arm curl, and compound rower.*

Lower Body and Torso

Leg Extension: Sit up-right on a leg extension machine. Be sure that your knees are in alignment with the axis of rotation. Select a weight that will allow you to fully extend your lower legs to 90-percent extension. Provide resistance on the downward motion. Repeat ten times. *Muscles used:* Quadriceps.

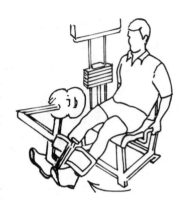

Leg Press: Assume a comfortable position in a leg press machine with feet shoulder-width apart. Slowly lower the weight down toward your body. Do not exceed a leg bend of 90 degrees. Keep the weight balanced equally between both feet. Repeat ten times. *Muscles used:* Thighs and hamstrings.

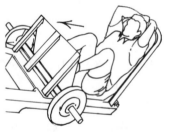

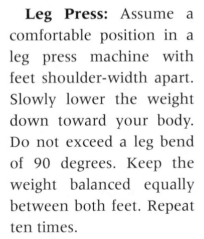

Leg Adduction: Sit comfortably in a leg adduction machine, being sure not to allow your legs to spread too far apart. Slowly bring your legs together by squeezing your inner thigh muscles. Slowly return to the starting position. (Abduction is optional.) Maintain good posture throughout the exercise. Repeat ten times.

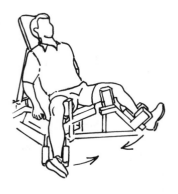

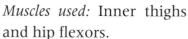

Muscles used: Inner thighs and hip flexors.

Abdominal Crunch: Sit comfortably in an abdominal crunch machine with your feet flat on the floor. Resting the crunch pad on your upper chest, press the pad toward your knees. Your lower body should remain stationary during the motion. Slowly return to the starting position. Repeat ten times.

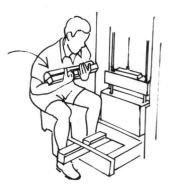

Muscles used: Abdominals and hip flexors.

Lower-back Extension: Sit comfortably in a lower back extension machine. Be sure that your feet are flat on the platform. Keeping your back straight, press the pad until you are in alignment with your lower body. Do not over extend. Control the weight on the return motion. Repeat ten times.
Muscles used: Lower and middle back.

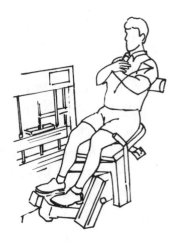

Rotary Torso: Sit upright on a rotary torso machine, interlocking your lower legs. Slowly rotate the pad, keeping your spine angle vertical. Slowly return the pad to the starting position. Repeat ten times on each side.
Muscles used: Oblique and middle back.

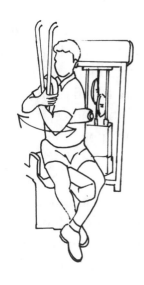

Special Note: Make a sensible choice from the exercises offered on the preceding pages. Do what will fit your time schedule, your fatigue level, and your personal goals. I have offered a number of different exercises so that you can choose the program to fit your situation and also have some variety. Mixing exercises that work the same area of the body has proven to be effective both developmentally and motivationally. Don't become overwhelmed by the number offered. You don't need to do many, but you do need to do some. Selecting a combination of strength, flexibility, and cardiovascular exercises that are mixed on alternate days and that take only twenty to forty-five minutes will make a noticeable difference within sixty days.

Endurance: Cardiovascular and Muscular

The casual pace of golf play does not make heavy endurance demands on the heart and lungs or cardiovascular system; nor does playing golf require intensive repetition (like making five hundred consecutive full swings), which would severely test one's muscular endurance. Nonetheless, golf does make enough demands on the body that endurance *definitely* becomes a factor when it comes to scoring.

Lack of endurance leads to fatigue, and fatigue is detrimental to performance in any skill activity. As one tires, balance is affected, along with speed, club control, even judgment and attention. Doing cardiovascular activities like fast walking, cycling or using a stationary exercise bike, jogging, swimming, stair climbing, even adding repetitions and sets to lighter-weight strength workouts can solve performance problems related to fatigue.

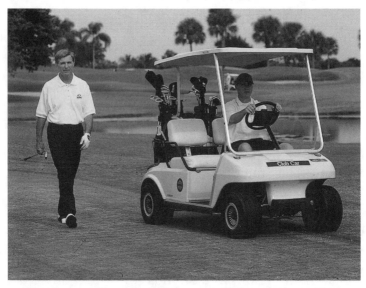

Having a golf car does not mean both people must ride.

The game of golf has built into it a program of cardiovascular fitness; it is called walking. Physicians worldwide extol the value of walking for fitness as a safe, reliable, and effective program. To take it out of the game by riding in a golf car is a health mistake. Golf cars are for people who would be unable to play otherwise due to a physical limitation and for the financial benefit of the facility renting them. Even when the golfer is confronted with the "required riding course" he or she may request that their companion drive or that they share the driving by walking alternate holes. You are not required to sit in the car for eighteen holes, only to rent it and return it. *The health benefits of golf, particularly those involving the cardiovascular and pulmonary systems, are reduced dramatically when the golf car is introduced.*

Built-In Fitness Activities

Much of one's success in any endeavor comes from the cultivation of good habits. Being in good physical condition is no exception. But a busy lifestyle unfortunately can turn intention to pretension. Fitness is not a "just pretend" condition. You can't buy it, borrow it, steal it, fake it, nor can you even store it for long. You must attend to it regularly and faithfully. One of the best ways for a busy person to accomplish this is with "built-ins," or fitness activities that you can insert into your daily life without requiring extra time. You do this by connecting them to activities you perform daily. Choose from the following list those you can fit into your lifestyle, or be creative and devise your own. *The secret is to make it convenient, regular, and above all a HABIT.*

Here are six activities around which you could choose to do "built-ins." Doing just one or two from each group should be adequate to produce results, both in your body and in your golf score.

Rise and Shine (Six "Built-Ins")

1. On waking, while in bed, pull your knees to your chest, gently stretching your lower back.

2. When putting on a shirt or blouse, raise one hand over a shoulder and slide it down your back. Push on that elbow with the opposite hand.

3. After putting on a pair of trousers, a skirt, or walking shorts, continue standing and cross one foot over the other and bend at the waist to reach toward the floor, touching it if possible; alternate legs.

4. When standing in front of the mirror, clasp your hands behind your lower back, and while bending forward, raise them as high as possible while the arms are extended. (See illustration.)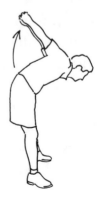

5. When putting on your shoes turn your head 90 degrees to the right, then left by gently pushing it with your hand: then hold ten seconds.

6. When finished dressing, get into a half-squat position with your back against the wall. Hold that position thirty to sixty seconds.

Note: What about getting up thirty minutes earlier and taking a brisk walk? That could be the best built-in habit of your life.

In the Bathroom (Six "Built-Ins")

1. Turn on the water. As it gets hot, do side bends, arms overhead and hands clasped.

2. As you lather your face to shave, or put on makeup, tighten your buttocks; hold as long as you can.

3. While shaving or fixing your hair, hold your abdomen in tight and count to fifty.

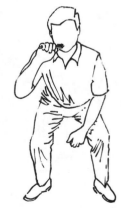

4. As you brush your teeth, do half squats from fifty to 100 reps; either single- or double-leg.

Half squats are easy to do while you brush your teeth.

5. When applying deodorant, do a single-arm reach toward the ceiling and rise on toes.

6. While putting on aftershave or facial lotion, raise and extend your leg, placing it on the vanity. Then reach forward to touch your toes and stretch your hamstrings. Repeat with the other leg.

Driving the Car (Six "Built-Ins")

1. At stoplights practice deep breathing, filling the lungs completely.

2. At stoplights grip the steering wheel as tightly as possible; release and repeat.

3. At stoplights lace your fingers in front of you, reverse their position, and stretch. Then return

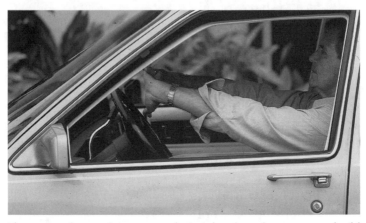

There are plenty of moments during the day when you can build exercises into your life, such as when you are driving the car.

them to the front, palms facing each other, and try to pull your hands apart with an isometric exercise.

4. While driving, do shoulder shrugs.

5. While driving, try abdominal isometrics, holding for thirty seconds.

6. While driving, carry a hand gripper and exercise each hand. (See illustration.)

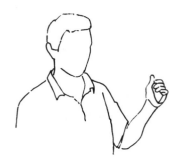

While Watching Television (Six "Built-Ins")

1. Ride a stationary bike, run on a treadmill, or jump rope.

2. Do bent-knee abdominal curl-ups.

3. Sit on the floor with one leg extended and with the other leg lying flat and bent to 90 degrees so that the foot touches the opposite knee. Reach your

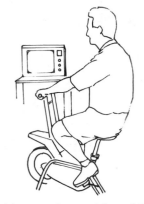

Ride a stationary bike while watching television.

hands toward the ankle of your extended leg and hold that position.

4. Lying on your back with both legs extended on the floor, alternately raise one leg to vertical, then swing it across your body until it touches the floor, so that it rotates and stretches your hips and trunk.

5. Grasp both knees and gently do tuck rolls on the carpet.

6. From a standing but spread-legged position, and while keeping your heels flat on the floor, lean forward until you make a bridge by placing your hands on the floor so you can look back through your extended legs (see picture on p. 20). Hold for thirty seconds.

At Work or Around the House (Six "Built-Ins")

Choose exercises from the previous lists that fit into your average day. You won't do all of these, but you will profit from doing *some* of them. Again, make up your own built-ins if necessary, but put them into your life until they become a habit. *There is so much wasted time in our lives that could be filled with productive fitness activities done on a very casual but regular basis.* Look for those opportunities. One helpful suggestion is to place home fitness products around the house where they are easy to see and convenient to use. A rubber tubing stretch device in a doorway, a hand gripper by the phone, a weighted club in a corner of the family room, or a learning aid such as this Power Swing Fan (see illustration), are all examples of giving yourself a chance to do more built-ins.

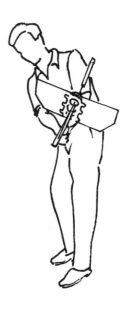

Other Considerations

Nutrition and Hydration

Even the best-conditioned athlete needs proper fuel, or food, for optimum performance. Seek to maintain your body weight within five pounds of when you felt you were at your top level of fitness. Maybe it was in high school or college and a long time ago, but it is a worthy goal. Eat those foods which over a lifetime of experience produce your best level of energy. The importance of low fat, moderate sugar and salt, and regular intake of water cannot be over emphasized. In fact, never pass a drinking fountain on the course without taking water. It has been demonstrated that a person can live for weeks without food but only days without water. *Water is the elixir of life,* transporting glucose and oxygen to the muscles, eliminating wastes, helping in digestion, cooling the body, and lubricating the joints. Drink eight glasses (64 oz.) in a normal day, more if exercising in hot temperatures. Don't wait until you are thirsty, because that is a sign that you are already liquid deficient, a factor in the deterioration of anyone's play.

Many players unknowingly give themselves the "halfway house blues" by stopping after nine holes for a soda, hot dog, and a candy bar. Stick to fruit, an energy bar, and water or juice. It takes some experimentation to find out which foods seem to work best before and/or during athletic performance, such as a round of golf. Some people can't handle solid foods when nervous and therefore prefer a liquid meal. Personally, I don't like to eat lunch just before playing a one o'clock competition. I focus on liquids and possibly an energy bar. And before an important event I would never introduce some new food to which I am unaccustomed. That is a time to definitely stick with what you know. What we do and don't eat has far greater influence on our state of health than we give credit. *Good nutrition advice abounds everywhere. Have enough willpower to abide by it.*

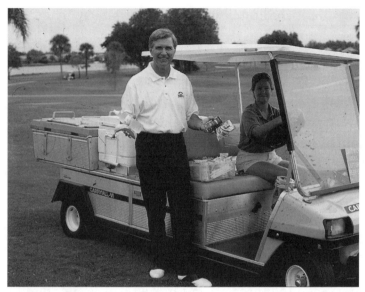

Finding good nutrition on the course is not always easy, but if a choice is available, water and fruit are better for you and your golf than soda and chips.

Injury and Surgery

Injury is always a possibility when adding more activity to your lifestyle. If you injure your body, don't make the mistake of ignoring the pain. *Listen to your body.* Give your body a chance to recover and don't rush getting back to your previous levels of weights or repetitions. This same counsel applies when you have had to suspend workouts for any reason, including illness, travel, or a busy schedule. Don't push it!

If pain occurs while you are doing a strength or flexibility exercise, stop. We are not talking here about fatigue, the "no pain, no gain" concept. If we want to make the most gain, we sometimes have to push ourselves beyond our comfort level. The pain we refer to here is a sharp pain signaling a potential injury. See your doctor if that kind of pain persists.

By far the most common mistake that golfers make after surgery, particularly seniors, is immediately attempting to match their previous activity level. For example, in hip replacement surgery the nerves in that area are cut more thoroughly than in some other locations like the knee, and the patient cannot feel when he is overstressing the joint. Too much load can lead to reinjury. So while it is important to work hard during rehabilitation, you must also be patient.

Rest

After strenuous physical activity the body needs rest to rejuvenate the cellular structure and muscular tissue and to replace energy reserves. That is why vigorous workout days are scheduled on alternate days with a day's rest in between. Stretching and light cardiovascular workouts can be done daily, but otherwise, include rest days.

Adequate sleep is often overlooked by the enthusiastic individual who has a busy lifestyle. If a commuter stays after work to exercise at the gym, comes home for a late dinner, spends time with the family, and catches up on the mail, news, and phone calls, it can be past midnight before the opportunity for sleep is available. If the morning alarm rings at 5:30 A.M. on a regular basis, he or she is probably not getting enough sleep.

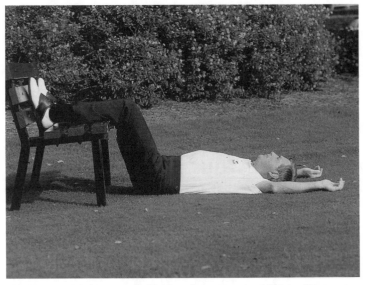

This is one of the most efficient short-term resting positions you can use.

Don't make the mistake of thinking you can make it up by "sleeping in" on the weekend. Your body develops a waking pattern that should be maintained. If you do need to catch up, go to bed earlier but keep your rising time close to normal. There is no correct set amount of sleep needed by every individual, but most adults require seven to eight hours in order to properly give their body and mind adequate rest. Experiment over a one-month period by modifying the amount you receive, monitoring it and determining which amounts of sleep make you feel the best. Getting the proper sleep or rest is vital to a strong mind and body, and hence performance on the golf course. That is the very reason why most touring professionals, even those in top condition, will not play more than three to four weeks in a row without taking a week off to rejuvenate both mind and body.

Protecting Your Back

Back problems can force a complete halt to your game. It's the most common cause of a golfer's physical "downtime." Don't risk injury to your back by reaching over to lift a heavy golf bag from a car trunk or bending over to pick the ball out of the hole while standing with your legs straight. Protect

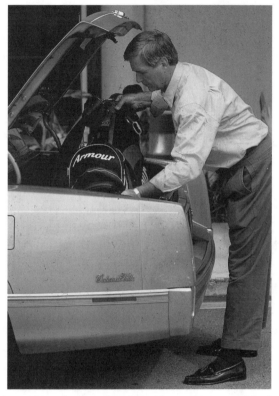

Danger! Reaching foreword to lift with your legs straight is a back killer. (I strained my back, which is normally strong, while posing for this picture.)

your back by building the strength and flexibility of the trunk region of your body, particularly the abdominal muscles. Combining this with stretching your hamstrings should help prevent back injury.

Conclusion

If you have wanted to improve your golf and your lifestyle by increasing your level of fitness but didn't know what to do, well now you do. There is no excuse. So don't wake up one day and say, "Gee, I wish I would have. . . ." JUST DO IT!

Note: If you are about to embark on a program suggested in this booklet, please check with your physician to see that your workout choice is appropriate. Start moderately when using weights or doing new exercises. Select a comfortable level of effort and progress gradually. **The biggest mistake made by those determined to start an exercise program is to push too hard for fast improvement. Be patient!**

Any reference to an exercise or training aid in this text can be fulfilled by calling Golf Around the World at 1-800-824-4279 or can be viewed at www.golfaroundtheworld.com.

Your Personal Golf Fitness Notes

Your Personal Golf Fitness Notes

Your Personal Golf Fitness Notes

Your Personal Golf Fitness Notes

Your Personal Golf Fitness Notes

Your Personal Golf Fitness Notes